Don't Be Alone in the Hospital

How to protect yourself from the risks inherent in hospitalization today.

By Bex Wylder, MD

To my girls, for their love, devotion and support

Table of Contents

Introduction

You've heard them hundreds of times on the radio. "Saint Joseph's Medical Center has the best cardiac surgeons and is the place for heart patients to get well". "At Mercy Hospital we care for more than your bones". "Cancer patients find a cure at Doctor's Medical Center of Hope".

The hospital marketing department and their consultants want you to believe that you should trust yourself completely to the employees, facilities, equipment, and Physicians at your local hospital.

But what about the horror stories you have heard from your aunt, or your friend in

Milwaukee, or seen in the newspaper about medical procedures or hospital stays gone horribly wrong?

How can you protect yourself from these circumstances when you must seek hospital care for your own illness, injury or surgery?

This book is intended to scare the daylights, and hopefully the complacency, out of you.

The stores here are real, the names, locations, and facilities have been removed or altered to protect me, your author, from the lawyers.

My own name above is a "nomme de plume" because I am a physician with several decades of working in a large tertiary care teaching hospital chain, and I still need my job. I can assure you, however, that the stories you are about to read are factual, and that the advice I have for prospective hospital patients is based on events I have personally witnessed or reviewed in official hospital meetings.

Please understand. Modern hospitals in the US employ truly amazing technology in medical and surgical care and can achieve what a few decades ago would have been regarded as miracles. Colon surgery through a half inch incision; reconstruction of bones, joints, ligaments, heart valves; transplants of hearts, lungs, kidneys, livers; high tech diagnostic and therapeutic tools that employ the latest in computer, optical, genetic, immunologic and drug technology; these would all be considered science fiction even 50 years ago.

At the same time, as you will see starting in a page or so, the dangers to you when you are in the hospital are greater than ever, and your need to plan for and protect yourself are likewise at an all time high.

That is what this book is for. This is not a book to help the medical profession or the hospital industry clean up its act. Others have written very eloquently on the subject. One of my favorites is "Internal Bleeding" by Dr. Robert Wachter. (Internal Bleeding: The Truth Behind America's

Terrifying Epidemic of Medical Mistakes, Robert M. Wachter and Kaveh G. Shojania)

This is also not a book on statistics. I will not bore you with tables of risk percentages for the accidents or injuries I relate. Yes, they are probably not very common, but if ONE of them happens to you or your relative when it could have been avoided by some fairly simple precautions, all the statistics in the world will not fix the injury or bring back your aunt, or make you feel any less grief.

This is a book for you with practical suggestions on protecting yourself from unintentional but potentially catastrophic injury or death from being in the hospital. I will relate some patient experiences to illustrate the types of precautions you need, and then discuss those precautions in more detail.

2. Jane Frey

Jane Frey was always the favorite visitor for her granddaughters, first because she brought them books, but mainly because she loved to ride her bicycle and the little girls thought that their bicycling granny was so cool.

Jane had always been active. She enjoyed good health for all of her life, and she paid attention to her diet. She had regular mammograms and she felt that her family doctor took good care of her on the rare occasions when she needed his assistance. Her husband has passed away 5 years before of heart disease, but she

13

enjoyed living alone and visiting her friends and relatives.

She particularly enjoyed bicycling, and always did at least 10 miles per day, even at 86 years old.

Then one day she slipped on a wet bathroom floor and broke her right hip.

That was embarrassing. Her daughter had tried to get some grippy mats for the house, but Jane just didn't like the way they looked or felt.

The injury was painful, of course, and she knew she needed to get the hip fixed so that she could continue being up and around and she hoped back on her bike in a few weeks or a month.

She had heard the radio ads for a local hospital's "Center of Excellence in Orthopedic surgery", and she felt reasonably happy with her doctor's recommendation that she have her surgery done there.

In fact, Jane's surgery went very well. There was minimal blood loss for the frequently bloody hip surgery. The surgeon had no difficulty with measuring, fitting, and installing the metal prosthesis into her right femur, and the operation was completed in only 90 minutes and Jane was off to recovery. Her vital signs were stable, with a pulse of 80, blood pressure of 120 over 80, and an oxygen saturation of 97%. The surgeon was happy with the result, and left orders for Jane to start getting up and putting weight on the leg by the next morning. At 10:00 on a Wednesday morning, Jane was moved to the "med-surg" ward to continue recovering.

Jane was by herself. Her daughters were working moms and had busy schedules. She didn't want to bother any of her other relatives or friends, and there was no one with her in the hospital.

Things at first seemed to be OK. Her vital signs were fairly stable. Her oxygen saturation had declined slightly to 95% but was still well within the normal range. Her pulse was still 85, and her blood pressure had declined slightly to 115 over 75.

The hospitalist who was responsible for her postoperative care saw her once about 11:00 am, and didn't notice any critical issues.

Over the course of the next several hours, however, Jane's condition started to gradually decline. Her blood pressure slipped lower, first to 100 over 70 then to 90 over 67, then to 88 over 62. Her pulse increased but not dramatically, first to 88 then to 95, and then to 110.

The most noticeable change was in her oxygen saturation, the number that indicates how much of the blood's oxygen carrying capacity is occupied by oxygen. This number declined from 95% to 90% then to 87%, 82% and 78%.

Jane wasn't awake, or easy to arouse for the first phase of the decline, and this was attributed to the pain medicine she had in her IV to control the surgical pain.

But as the day wore on, she became more agitated, and began thrashing her arms. At this point, her nurse asked for an order for restraints, and Jane's arms were placed in padded cuffs that were tied to the bed rails with their attached straps.

The nurse also increased the flow rate of her IV, so that she could receive more pain medicine.

There were no other nursing notes to indicate that there was a problem with Jane's condition.

At 9:00 pm, the nursing shift changed, and a new nurse took over Jane's care. In the nursing "report" session, the only mention of Jane was that she was the "post-op Hip in 441A".

The nurse who came on eventually reached Jane's room as she rounded on her patients for the start of the shift. By this time, Jane had a pulse of 120, a blood pressure of 75 over 50, and an oxygen saturation of 78%. Although there had been no mention of Jane having a problem during report, the new nurse was concerned, and after Jane continued to have critically low vital signs called for the "ACT team" to evaluate Jane. The "Rapid Response Team" (RRT) or "Acute Care

Team" (ACT team) is a panel of doctors and nurses that are organized in many hospitals to respond to patients who have not stopped their breathing or heart rate (and who need a "Code Blue" for resuscitation) but who have had a change in condition and need more intensive evaluation than the floor nurse, who has several other patients to take care of, can provide.

The ACT team assessed Jane, and concluded that she was basically in shock. She was hypotensive (low blood pressure); tachycardic (rapid heart rate) and desaturating (low oxygen saturation) and the condition had been severe and deteriorating for hours.

Jane was transferred to ICU, intubated, placed on a mechanical ventilator, given oxygen, medicines to increase her blood pressure ("pressors") and increased intravenous fluids. Unfortunately, she had suffered irreversible brain damage, and later the next day instead of starting to walk up and down the hall, her daughters decided to "turn off the machine" and Jane was pronounced dead. A routine hip surgery on an elderly but otherwise healthy patient ended with a fatal result.

The nurse responsible for taking care of Jane after her surgery had basically just watched her deteriorate over more than 10 hours without alerting the doctor, calling for a supervisor to help, calling the ACT team or doing anything other than tying Jane to the bed so that she wouldn't move around. Why? We don't know what the nurse was thinking. She was promptly fired from the hospital. The case was entered into the "risk management" and "peer review" processes. These are the mechanisms in the hospital for studying "adverse outcomes" both to evaluate need for improvement in processes, and to assess and manage the potential for patients or families to seek damages for malpractice.

There was no reason that Jane had to die in the hospital. Although elderly, she was in good mental and physical health, and "her operation was a success".

What Jane lacked, and what you need, was someone to watch over her while she could not watch over herself in the hospital.

3. Protecting yourself when you have surgery

You can take simple precautions to protect yourself from harm when you are in the hospital for surgery.

You need to have mature, attentive, relatives or friends with you in the pre-op and recovery phases to avoid unnecessary misfortune like Jane's. They are your advocates.

The first thing to understand is that with some exceptions (mainly in obstetrical deliveries) relatives or friends are prohibited from being present in the operating room during your surgery. This is a reasonable rule that is for the protection of the patient, the surgery personnel, and the potential visitors. Operating rooms are busy places with many pieces of equipment, with need for sterility, and with multiple doctors, nurses, and technicians providing for the patient's anesthesia, the operation, the instruments and equipment, the various video and other monitors, and sometimes even the robotic control system. They are not places conducive to visitors. They are also, for the most part, not the part of the hospital where the patient is at the greatest risk.

There are four basic types of potential problems in surgery, and for three of them, you can improve your odds by having an advocate with you.

The first type of surgical problem, and the one that your advocate can do nothing about, is the problem during the operation.

Even having general anesthesia without an incision has a small risk of death or injury. Sometimes the anesthesiologist will damage or dislodge one of your teeth. Sometimes the way your body is positioned or arranged can potentially lead to nerve damage. Sometimes people's hearts stop on the table and they can't get them started again.

Rarely, things go wrong during the surgery itself. The surgeon can cut the wrong blood vessel, nerve, or piece of bowel. There may be damage to a ureter, one of the tubes connecting the kidney and the bladder, or there may be bleeding that is difficult or impossible to control. Most of these issues are promptly recognized and dealt with. Your best (or maybe only) protection from these problems is to find a surgeon who is well regarded in the community and who can communicate with you in a way that you can understand.

Among the problems that your advocate can help with there are three main types.

The first problem to avoid is so called "wrong site surgery". You came in for a right hip fracture, and you want to make sure that the operation is conducted on your right hip, not the normal left one. The worst examples of this error have included amputating the healthy leg and leaving the diseased one or taking out the healthy kidney and leaving the one with cancer in.

Most hospitals have instituted "mark your site" programs where the patient and doctor participate in making a mark with a pen on the part of the body to be operated on. You and your advocate need to make sure that the surgeon and the nurses don't forget this step. You both can be sure that the site marking happens, and that the correct part or side of the body is marked. Inside the operating room, the surgical team should conduct a "timeout" before the operation to again assure that the operation is happening on the correct body part.

The second problem, and the one that affected our friend Jane, is the issue of post-operative monitoring. Although there was not an autopsy and we do not know for sure the reasons why, Jane's vital signs began to deteriorate after she was moved to the ward, and her incompetent nurse either didn't pay attention to the deteriorating vital signs or did not react appropriately when there would still have been time to save Jane's life. The most egregious error, in the view of some who reviewed the case, was the failure to carefully assess Jane's condition before tying her to the bed (or putting her in restraints, as they would say in hospital-speak).

Jane's deterioration may have been for several reasons.

She may have had internal bleeding from the surgical site or from another site.

She may have become dehydrated through incorrect management of her IV fluids,

She may have had a pre-existing heart condition that was not detected prior to surgery, or she may have had a reaction to one of the medications used in anesthesia or for pain.

Had she had a friend or relative watching her parameters, especially her oxygen saturation (which is usually displayed on a monitor right by the bedside) her advocate could have insisted on an earlier intervention, demanded to speak to the nursing supervisor, or even phoned Jane's doctors to insist that she be evaluated. If there had been an intervention after an hour or two instead of about 10 ours, Jane might be with us today, riding her bicycle with her new hip, and bringing books to the granddaughters again.

The last kind of problem that can happen after surgery regards the issue of general medical care, medications, and their proper administration and dosage. This issue will be the subject of the next couple of chapters.

4. June Boyer

June Boyer was ill, but she didn't need to die in the hospital.

She was 74 years old, and she had been admitted for trouble breathing. She had a history of lung problems, and had some problems with an irregular heart beat called atrial fibrillation, where the atrial part of the heart beats at a rapid rate not coordinated with the ventricles.

Anyway, she had been admitted to the hospital and was under the care of a hospitalist, a physician trained in internal medicine who specializes in caring for patients in the hospital.

Dr. G, her physician, was off for a weekend, and he had arranged for Dr. S to cover for him. When Dr. S. saw June, he noted her atrial fibrillation and decided to start her on blood thinners, to avoid the potential (increased in atrial fib patients) of blood clots and stroke. The medicine that Dr. S. prescribed was Coumadin, also known by the generic name Warfarin. When warfarin is used, it is necessary for the patient's clotting times to be monitored to assure that the dose is neither too much nor too little, and the monitoring is done with a laboratory test called a "prothrombin time" or "protime" for short. But Dr. S didn't order a protime. He later testified that he thought the test was automatically ordered, but it was not.

On Monday Dr. G returned and resumed care of June. There was no documentation that Dr. S had mentioned the start of warfarin therapy in their "handoff" of the patient. There is no evidence that Dr. G noticed the addition of warfarin to the medication list when he reviewed June's chart on Monday.

On Tuesday, after June had been on warfarin for 4 days, the pharmacist wrote a note in her chart suggesting to Dr. G that he order a protime to check on the warfarin dose. Either Dr. G did not see the note, or he ignored it. No protime was ordered, and warfarin was continued. Nurses administered the warfarin dose each day and did not ask the pharmacy why a protime wasn't done. Later, a nurse observed that many employees of the hospital were reluctant to call Dr. G. because he often became disagreeable, hostile, and belligerent when he perceived them to be questioning his medical judgment.

June continued to be in the hospital for another week under Dr. G's care. On day 11 of warfarin therapy, she was noted to be bleeding from her gums and from puncture sites where blood had been drawn. A prothrombin time was finally ordered, and her clotting time was increased far beyond the desired therapeutic range for warfarin therapy. Treatment to reverse the effect of warfarin was started, but June developed a severe stroke that was documented on CT scan to result from a massive intracerebral bleed. She expired the next day. Her bleeding episode was caused by the complete loss of normal blood clotting function due to warfarin treatment in combination with other drugs she was also receiving. The interaction would have been detected if there had been appropriate monitoring of her protime, but neither of her physicians or pharmacists ever ordered a protime.

The hospital, and later the state medical board investigated this case. Many procedural changes were put in place in an attempt to prevent future events of this type.

5. Protecting yourself when you're sick

If June had been accompanied by a relative who was paying attention, and if they had asked about the medicines she was being given and the need for monitoring of blood thinners, the inattention or incompetence of the physicians, nurses, and pharmacists taking care of her could perhaps have been prevented from resulting in her premature demise.

Many patients who are familiar with the hospital environment, often because they work in the hospital as doctors, nurses, laboratory techs etc., relate the experience of having nurses attempt to give them medications that had not been ordered by their physicians.

Your patient advocate needs to know what medications you are supposed to be on, and needs to challenge those administering medications to assure that they are the ones that are supposed to be given, and also the dose and timing of the medicine. Whether it is the wrong bed, the wrong room, or someone with a similar name, you don't want to be receiving medications intended for someone else.

In June's case, the issue is a little more complicated. Blood thinners or "anticoagulant medications" such as warfarin can be life saving, but unless monitored carefully they can also be life taking as in June's case. Your advocate needs to make sure that if you are given blood thinners, especially warfarin, that your clotting times are checked regularly.

Although initial recovery from many types of surgery, as in chapter 3, can usually be accomplished within a day or two, or even less as many laparoscopic surgeries are done as outpatients, when you are in the hospital for an illness, or a more major surgery, you may end up staying for a week or more. This brings up a new dimension to the need for a patient advocate since one person cannot be expected to be awake and vigilant for days at a time. You will need to have more than one person willing to take shifts so that oversight and advocacy for you can be available at all times. Just because it is the middle of the night in the hospital does not mean that you are immune from receiving the wrong medication or being summoned for someone else's procedure.

6. Mark Fisher

Mark Fisher was a disabled 45 year old who came to the hospital for a gallbladder operation. He had been having pains in his abdomen and the films had shown gallstones. Unfortunately, after he was admitted, he had some upper gastrointestinal distress, and the surgery was delayed for awhile so that he could recover. More unfortunately, he never got to surgery.

Besides his gallbladder problem, Mark suffered from anemia, or low blood hemoglobin. His hemoglobin level was running around 8.5 grams per 100 ml of blood, while a normal male would be between 14 and 18. One morning, his routine hemoglobin check came back at 4.5 instead of 8.5. He was also having a faster pulse rate, and his "stomach trouble" seemed worse.

The nurse noticed these changes, so she called Mark's doctor, Dr. M.

Dr. M. must have been busy seeing his patients at his office or at another hospital, because he didn't call back right away. In fact he didn't call back for more than 90 minutes. In the meantime, the lab had repeated the blood count on Mark's sample and had confirmed that he had had a major drop in his blood count since the day before. The nurse checked on Mark occasionally, but otherwise kept waiting for Dr. M. to call.

At about 2 hours after she had called Dr. M. another physician was in the area, and the nurse asked him to check on Mark. He did, and he was able to pronounce Mark dead.

Mark Fisher died of bleeding into his stomach and small intestine from a bleeding ulcer. An ulcer in his stomach lining had eroded into a small artery, and he had started bleeding into the stomach. The blood was carried downstream in the GI tract to the small intestine, and when the autopsy was done, the stomach and upper small intestine were full of blood. Mark bled to death in the hospital.

The nurse recognized that something was wrong; a big drop in blood count can indicate that there has been internal bleeding. She took action, paging Dr. M., but when he didn't call back promptly, or for more than an hour and a half she didn't do anything else.

What could she have done?

Well, after that incident, among others, the hospital instituted their "ACT team". As discussed earlier, this team is prepared to respond to a patient whose condition has deteriorated or become unstable and who needs a more intensive assessment.

She could have used the "chain of command".   Nursing departments are organized in a somewhat hierarchical fashion, with head nurses supervising floor nurses, and "house supervisors" in charge of the entire hospital. When a nurse has a problem, like not being able to reach the doctor for a crashing patient, she can ask for help or intervention from her higher ups.

Mark, like our prior patients, was alone in the hospital, and therefore defenseless from the lack of prompt attention to his medical needs.

Although there are never any guarantees of survival, if Mark's condition had been promptly assessed, he could have received additional IV fluids, blood transfusion, "upper GI endoscopy" to assess his condition, a CT scan, or even emergency surgery. After all, he was IN THE HOSPITAL, a place that has doctors and nurses whose job is to take care of your health.

Could an advocate or companion have speeded up the process? Most certainly.

Some hospitals now have instituted a "Code H". This is a system allowing family members to express their concerns directly to the facility when they have a problem with the care being delivered or a concern regarding a specific issue. Would a Code H in Marks case have allowed him to survive?

There's no way to know for sure, but simply allowing him to keep bleeding into his stomach for over 2 hours was certainly unlikely to help his chances.

7. Protecting Yourself from Abandonment

Although Mark's nurse realized that something was seriously wrong with Mark's lab values, and make at least a token attempt to intervene by calling his doctor, at the end of the day Mark was abandoned by the hospital for the two hours between the recognition of the problem and his death.

If you are the patient's advocate, you need to learn about your options for escalating concerns about the person you are advocating for to "the management", and doing so in a timely fashion. It is not going to help your friend or relative when you complain to the hospital CEO or file a malpractice suit after they die. If you are more interested in the financial settlement than the company of your friend of relative, ask them to find someone else to be their advocate.

This is one of the most challenging roles for the patient advocate. Everyone has heard the tales of patients waiting a long time for the nurse to respond to the "call light" when they want to ask for some more ice chips, or any other routine concern.

Most of the time the delay was annoying or perhaps uncomfortable but not life threatening.

In cases like Mark's every minute counted.

Fortunately, at present, larger hospitals have experienced internal medicine physicians physically present in the hospital 24/7. This provides an important resource for patients whose condition deteriorates. Until a few years ago, the only physicians reliably in the hospital would be the emergency room physicians, other physicians "rounding" on their patients, or surgeons engaged in performing surgery in the OR's.

Being aware of the hospitalist system in your hospital could be an important piece of information for your advocate. Being vigilant regarding significant changes in their condition and insisting on timely assessment and intervention can be critical.

8. Keith Sutherland/Keith Miller

Keith Miller's story has a happy ending, but it also illustrates a critical part of the patient advocate's task.

Keith was in the hospital for his back pain, and was scheduled for a disk operation the next day. In the afternoon, a student nurse came into his room, 221B, with some blood tubes and a tourniquet, and announced that the doctor had asked for blood to be drawn for lab tests. Keith never enjoyed these sessions, because he had always had "small veins" and they usually ended up poking him two or three times before they got their sample, but he assumed that the doctor had a good reason for wanting another blood sample.

In fact, the blood order that day was for another Keith, Keith Sutherland, who was in room 231A on the same ward. The student nurse addressed him as Keith, but never checked his hospital arm band to confirm his identity. She was also unable to obtain any blood from his left arm, that was the good vein, after two tries, and she then called for her supervising RN to take over. The supervising RN came in and checked Keith's arms for veins, and was able to obtain a sample from his right arm. She also failed to check his armband.

As a result, a sample from Keith Miller, who is blood type A, was drawn and labeled with the Name Keith Sutherland, who is blood type O, and sent to the laboratory for cross matching.

After the blood was tested, and the blood units for transfusion were selected, the doctor for Keith Sutherland ordered the transfusion of one unit of blood.

People with type O blood have natural antibodies that react with type A cells and will break them down and remove them from the circulation. Transfusion of "incompatible blood" can have serious consequences, and may be fatal to the recipient. The most common cause of fatal hemolytic transfusion reaction is "clerical error".

Later that day, another nurse started the transfusion on Keith Sutherland. He was in the hospital for some severe rectal bleeding and his doctor had ordered a transfusion to aid in his recovery. Within a few minutes after the blood was started into his vein, he experienced some back pain that he reported to the nurse. Fortunately, she was paying attention to the protocol for transfusions, and she stopped the infusion of blood after only a few cc's had been transfused. Also fortunately, Keith Sutherland was awake and not under anesthesia in surgery, or otherwise unable to promptly report his symptoms and get the incompatible transfusion stopped.

At that point, the error was discovered, and the transfusion cancelled. Luckily, having received only 10 or 15 ccs of the wrong blood, Keith Sutherland recovered completely without major symptoms or damage.

A "root cause analysis" was done by the risk management department revealing the problem with the sample collection and labeling.

Shortly thereafter, his hospital adopted a new practice in blood transfusions. Now they require two separate tests for blood type from different samples before they give blood to a patient except in the most extreme emergencies, and in those cases they generally give "O negative" blood that is compatible with any recipient. Other hospitals have a special arm band that is placed only when a sample for blood transfusion is collected. Both systems are designed to avoid errors like in this case where a mis labeled sample exposed a patient to a potentially fatal transfusion reaction.

What is the message for the patient advocate? Make sure that anyone collecting a sample, administering medication, or performing any other service on your friend or relative has correctly identified them by their wrist band prior to either obtaining the

sample or giving the medicine or treatment.

9. Protecting Yourself From Identification Error

With the wide variety of deeply invasive and potentially hazardous procedures going on in a large hospital every day, some of the most tragic errors occur when the wrong patient is selected for the planned procedure. At the very beginning of a hospital stay, every patient receives a wrist band to identify them to the system. The first priority is to make sure that when they place the wrist band on the patient that it has the correct name and information.

One of the habits that have led to patient misidentification is the practice of some nurses of referring to patients primarily by their room and bed number, "The patient in 331B" or just "331B" as opposed to their name. Sometimes the patients get moved around without the nurses' knowing about it.

In the case of laboratory samples in particular, the required protocol is for the nurse or phlebotomist to label the samples while they are at the bedside in the presence of the patient and after checking the wristband. The further away the sample travels from the patient before it is labeled, usually in someone's pocket, the more likely it is to end up with an incorrect label. Make sure that the person drawing blood from your relative does not put it in their pocket or onto a tray without it being labeled correctly.

Some hospitals now use hand held bar code scanners to verify the correct patient and sample identification. They can scan the patient's armband and the blood tubes and verify a match, or in some cases they print the labels at the bedside at the time of the draw.

Whatever the technology used for patient identification; the basics are as always the most important. The hospital staff must verify the patient's identification before every sample is obtained, medication is given, or procedure is started.

One account from Dr. Wachter's "Internal Bleeding" regarded an elderly female patient who was brought from her room to the Cardiac Catheterization laboratory for an invasive procedure. Despite the fact that there were 17 (yes, seventeen) opportunities to check her identification and to determine that she was not the patient for whom the procedure was intended, she was saved at only the last second from an unnecessary and potentially dangerous procedure that she did not need.

10. Other ways to protect yourself

So you may be saying to yourself,"I don't know who to call to be my advocate, my kids are all busy with work, they might lose their job if they have to spend a week in the hospital babysitting me, and the grandkids are too busy playing video games or smoking pot to spend time protecting their cranky old Grandpa; plus I just don't want to be a bother".

Well, there are other alternatives to find someone to help you navigate the hospital and medical system and to be your advocate.

First of all, discuss the issue with your friends, especially the retired ones. You can certainly offer a reciprocal arrangement, where you will advocate for them if they will for you. Besides the several specific issues outlined above, having another person with you to listen to what the doctor or nurse is saying and help get the questions asked can be incredibly valuable. Experienced nurses find that the most common questions patients ask after a visit from their doctor in the hospital is "what did he say anyway?" .

Serving as an advocate for someone else who is going to the hospital is a great way to increase your own understanding of the need for patient advocates and also of the types of concerns that might arise in your own hospitalization.

Whether you are working with family or friends, you will want to start preparing them for advocate duty by reviewing the checklist from appendix A. That will also help you to know that they have the right preparation to be taking care of you when you may be either medicated or exhausted from the hospital experience. Planning is easier when you are scheduled for elective surgery or hospitalization. It is more difficult to arrange for when you have an emergency admission or procedure, but that further emphasizes the need for advance planning.

If you are completely alone in the world, if your friends and family are either not available or unwilling, or if you don't have confidence in friends or family, a growing number of services are being established to provide patient advocacy just as we describe above.   These services are often started by retired nurses, and an advantage is that they have a thorough knowledge of how hospitals work and of how to navigate the system, as well as good familiarity with the vocabulary of nurses and doctors so that they can translate for you when necessary.

In addition to protecting you in the hospital, these services can assist with outpatient care, second opinions, insurance issues, care planning, and many aspects of your health care.

You can also arrange to hire your own private duty nurse. This individual can be available to assure that you or your relative receives the attention and the freedom from misadventure that they need.

Training or educational programs are also now available to train patient advocates, and it is one of the newest career options in health care.

11. Why are Hospitals so dangerous?

The large majority of patients who come to the hospital for surgery or medical care have a successful course and return home, but several factors have contributed in the past few years to increased potential for injury or death.

a.   Hospital patients are sicker.

First, both the hospitals and especially the medical payment apparatus (that is insurance companies and the governments) have contributed to making hospital stays shorter and to keeping many people who would have been hospitalized 40 or 50 years ago out of the hospital altogether. Some of the reasons are due to technology. In the "old days" if you had surgery for your appendix you could expect to be in the hospital for a week. Now, that operation is usually done on an outpatient basis using the laparoscope, a tube with a fiber optic video camera that allows the surgeon to examine and operate on your appendix through a tiny incision next to your navel. Due to the very limited trauma to the abdominal wall, and to the more limited time under anesthesia, there is not a need to stay overnight.

Other reasons for shorter stays are that hospitals and payers (that's the insurance and government again) constantly monitor "length of stay" statistics, and there is a growing practice where the hospital is penalized financially when a patient stays longer than the "standard length of stay" for whatever illness or surgery they have.

Even patients who need prolonged inpatient care are often transferred to an "extended care facility" if they need a more prolonged period of recovery or rehabilitation after their illness or surgery.

Given our examples, staying in the hospital for a shorter duration is a good thing, but the side effect is that the people who are in the hospital now are considerably sicker than they were a few decades ago.

This means that the complexity of their care, the medicines that they receive, and the diagnostic studies they undergo, and even the surgical options are all more varied and more potent than they used to be, the nurses and doctors have a more stressful and demanding environment, and inevitably the potential for misapplication of these drugs or procedures can lead to greater harm.

b. Technology

Technologies can be life saving and labor saving, but they have their downsides as well. Let's see a few examples.

50 years ago when you had an intravenous infusion, the rate could only be determined by a nurse or a pharmacist counting the number of drops per minute going into the IV.

Now, the hospital uses programmable infusion pumps to meter and regulate the delivery of an intravenous solution. While they are easier to program than your VCR clock (and if you don't understand that reference you have a few years before you should need this book), now the nurse has to know not only how to count drops per minute but also how to program a fairly complicated computer controlled device that will deliver the medication into your vein through an IV line using a pump. As with any type of technology, there is a potential for error. The pump manufacturers realized this, and they installed some electronic "guard rails" in the software for their instrument to avoid improper programming, but even the guard rails are not always effective.

One patient, Alex Finch, was receiving a chemotherapy drug for their colon cancer. The plan was to infuse the bag of medicine over a 12 hour period. This schedule would give the medicine a chance to work on the cancer for an extended period of time and would limit the damage to Alex's normal tissues at the same time. Due to an error in pump programming, the medicine was infused over only 45 minutes. Alex died the next day, basically poisoned by the too-rapid delivery of a powerful drug that was given to cure his cancer and save his life.

A few years ago, the news reported a mishap involving the programming of a radiation therapy machine. These machines are elaborate, multi-million dollar pieces of equipment using linear accelerator technology to produce beams of radiation that are directed at cancerous tumors using sophisticated dosimetry software and computers. Progress in radiation therapy has significantly improved medicine's ability to control or even cure certain cancers. This patient's system was programmed incorrectly, and as a result they received a much higher than intended dose of radiation to their chest. The result was a severe injury to their spinal cord and they became a paraplegic.

Within the past 6 months, calibration on a CT scanner was inadvertently set to the wrong value. As a result several patients received excessive radiation to their bodies, and at least one has linear stripes of hair loss on their scalp at about 4 mm spacing, corresponding to the "slices" of radiation delivered by the CT.

c. Computers

Another cause of hospital risk is the computer information systems that are now used in almost every hospital to keep track of the care.

George Fern was a patient who was on dialysis for his chronic renal failure. He came to the emergency room of a large hospital because of some nausea and vomiting. He arrived at about 10pm one evening. Some initial laboratory tests were ordered, and the patient was admitted to the floor. His doctor ordered some "AM labs", thinking that they would be drawn and tested the next morning, now about 6 hours away. What he didn't realize was that after 1:00 am in that hospital, orders for "AM labs" were interpreted to be for the next day, about 30 hours away, and not the same day, but later in the morning. As a result, no follow up orders were entered. It was also the intention of the ED physician to refer George to a nephrologist, a specialist in kidney disease, to check on the status of his kidney disease and his dialysis, but that referral never happened. With renal failure and without dialysis, George's potassium level became elevated. Ultimately, almost 24 hours after he first came to the hospital, he suffered from cardiac arrest and died. His potassium was finally checked while he was in a Code Blue, and it was almost 7, a dangerously high level. Was the delayed lab value responsible for George's death?

Probably not by itself, but it might have prompted his doctors or nurses to pay more attention to him than they did.

Angie Bowden was a 28 year old female who came to the hospital with abdominal pain. Due to a new software program for managing radiology images, the abdominal CT scan from a different patient was accidentally placed under her name. The radiology tech noticed the error, but didn't succeed in correcting it, and the other patient's scan remained in her file and was read by the radiologist. Unfortunately for Angie, the other patient had a 4 inch tumor on one of his kidneys. Thanks to the misfiling of the electronic films, Angie had one of her normal kidneys removed. The hospital settled the case for $2 million, but that will not replace Angie's kidney.

Another issue with the computer medical record carried over from the paper record. There may be a single piece of information buried in a 4 or 5 inch chart that will make all the difference in the drug therapy, treatment, or surgery planned for the patient. In the paper chart, sometimes the physician who needed to know that piece of information was not aware of it because it was simply "buried". Computers have the potential to make information more readily available. For example more than one person can be looking at the electronic chart at the same time. Computer "charts" are also voluminous and challenging to navigate, however, and there is still the potential, and sometimes the reality that the information needed to avoid a disastrous outcome was "buried".

d. Nursing care

Another reason for patient risks in hospitals is more controversial and politically charged, and that is nursing care.

Although one of the recent trends in hospital care has been for the hospital to contract with "hospitalist physicians" to provide continuous in house physician care for their patients, the floor nurse is still the individual with by far the most patient contact and responsibility for monitoring hospital patients.

A good and experienced nurse can certainly provide the margin between health and disaster for a patient who takes a turn for the worse in the hospital. Likewise, an inattentive or incompetent nurse can be a disaster.

Over the course of the last 20 years, and especially before the 2008 economic crash, nursing shortages were the rule of the day in hospitals. This resulted in several trends, including significantly increased levels of nursing salaries and also in creative and aggressive strategies to recruit new nurses to hospital staffs. One of the ways that hospitals use to fill their vacancies was to contract with so called "traveler agencies". These companies employ nurses who prefer to work for 3 to 6 month rotations in different parts of the state or country rather than having a single location. The cost to the hospital is about double the cost of hiring a nurse as a full time employee, but some hospitals have been unable to provide needed staffing levels any other way, and some larger hospitals have more than 100 "traveler nurses" working at any one time. Many traveler nurses are very competent and diligent. Hospital operations, especially information systems, vary considerably from hospital to hospital, and there is a considerable "learning curve" when a new employee arrives. It is also probable that the traveler nurse has a lower level of interest or commitment in the hospital or patients in a location where they expect to work for only 5 or 6 months, and where none of their friends or family resides.

In any case, I have seen several instances when a traveler nurse was responsible for failing to adequately take care of a patient with disastrous consequences.

Another hospital strategy for filling nursing positions has been to aggressively recruit from other countries, particularly Canada, the Philippines, the UK, and India. Many immigrant nurses provide excellent care and have good English skills. Others may be more marginal, either in their training, experience, or command of the language.

The other concern that has been illustrated recently is that the nurses' job has become progressively more technology intensive. This may be a good thing when technologies relieve some of the burden of work by automatically recording and displaying vital signs, or even sounding alarms when things went out of bounds. It can be a bad thing when nurses are not able to master the skills needed to function effectively in their technology rich environment. Programming IV pumps is just such an issue, as illustrated above.

e. Resident Hour Restrictions

Residency training programs, in which physicians are trained to practice their selected specialty after they finish medical school and receive their MD or DO degree, have changed drastically within the past decade. Following some tragic and very high profile cases (look up Libby Zion) where severe patient injury or death was attributed to either fatigued resident physicians or lack of faculty supervision, the organizations responsible for accrediting programs have instituted dramatic changes in the hours that residents can work per week, per day, and per shift. While there may be benefits from these changes, one consequence has been found to be of potential harm to patients, and that is the increased number of "handoffs" occurring in a patient's care.

Every time there is a shift change, whether of nurses, hospitalist physicians, or residents, there is the necessity for informing the new crew about the events of the past shift. This is called the "handoff". While sleep deprived residents may cause errors or omissions, it is also true that more "handoffs", as created by the resident hour restrictions, cause more errors as well.

Your advocate needs to make sure that issues involving your friend or relative are not "lost in translation" or missed in the shift change of nurses or doctors.

12. Other resources

Books

- **Internal Bleeding: The Truth Behind America's Terrifying Epidemic of Medical Mistakes Robert M. Wachter , Kaveh G. Shojania May 10, 2005.**

- **To Err is Human: Building a Safer Health System, Institute of Medicine Consensus report, November 1, 1999**

- **Critical Conditions: the Essential Hospital Guide to Get Your Loved One out Alive, M Erenclou, 2008**

Web Sites

- http://www.nyp.org/glossary/index

  for common medical terms used in health care

- http://www.mayoclinic.com

Medical conditions and illnesses

- http://www.webMD.com

- http://www.merck.com

- http://www.medlineplus.gov

- http://www.healthfinder.gov

- http://www.cdc.gov

- http://www.HHS.gov

- http://www.NIH.gov

- http://www.ismp.org

  Institute for Safe Medication Practices

- http://www.jcipatientsafety.org

  The Joint Commission's Center for Patient Safety

- http://www.carepages.com

Patient and Family support

- http://www.healthgrades.com

  Hospital and Nursing Home rankings

- http://www.nursingworld.com
- http://www.jointcommission.org

Appendix A – A checklist for you and your patient advocate

Before you go to the hospital

- **Check on your "Advance directives" do you want full resuscitation if your heart stops?**

- **Check on your medical power of attorney you may need this to allow your advocate to see your information and be able to stay with you.**

- **Check on your current medications, and take a legible list, don't just gather up all the old medicine bottles you have lying around.**

- Make a list of your allergies, your blood type, and of any other important previous health issues (especially things like metal implants, pacemakers, prior surgeries, bleeding problems, etc).

- Understand the procedure or surgery you are planned to have and educate yourself on the possible adverse outcomes.

- Select your advocate (or advocates if you face more than a brief stay.)

- If you do not have a friend or family member, consider an advocate service or a private duty nurse.

- Review the items below with them to be sure they understand your wishes and some of the key terms and issues. This may be a longer or shorter task depending on their level of education and familiarity with the health care system.

- Consult your hospital's information number regarding your ability to have your advocate in the room with you at all times other than when you are in surgery (or possibly intensive care). Many hospitals are moving to mostly or all private rooms, and these rooms often have space and either chairs or beds to allow a family member or other advocate to stay in your room with you. Verify their policy before you head to the hospital. You do not want your advocate to be excluded from your room outside of "visiting hours".

- Confirm the hospital's policy on "Code H" or other options for family members or other advocates to get additional attention for the patient.

- Make sure that your doctor (if you are going in for surgery) gives you an expected length of stay and that you understand exactly what kind of procedure you are planned to have

- Follow any bathing or cleaning directions from the hospital or physician. Some hospitals have directions for how to clean your skin prior to checking in for elective surgery.

- Be sure to bring along any items you need for your comfort, entertainment, and safety. These may include snacks, books, magazines, music players, electronic books, etc. Be sure that you have a list of items that you take along.

- Anticipate any language, specific dietary, or cultural issues with the patient and prepare a list for the hospital

On Arriving At the Hospital

- Be sure that the identity band placed on your wrist in admitting contains an accurate version of your information, particularly your name.

- If you have a common name (like John Smith, Vang Nguyen, or Maria Gonzales) be sure that the hospital tags you with a "common name alert".

- Be sure that your allergies are updated and correct in the hospital records at admission. If you have a severe drug or food allergy be sure that your chart is marked on the cover to indicate this issue. If you are at an "all electronic" hospital be sure that the computer contains the needed information on allergies and their severity.

- **Verify that your advocate will be able to accompany you to your room and through as much of your care experience as physically possible.**

- **Review the patient's specific language, dietary, and cultural issues with the admissions personnel to assure that they are entered in the patient's record.**

In Your Room

- **Alert the nurses and other staff caring for you to the presence of your advocate and their role in protecting you. It is not necessary to be overly suspicious of the staff. Just clearly indicate who your advocate is and that they have your permission to access any of your information and to question anyone providing services to you in the hospital. You certainly want to start out in a friendly and cooperative way with your nurses and other personnel.**

- You and your advocate need to get to know your primary nurse, to understand the hospital's nursing shifts, and to know how to call additional resources if necessary. You will want to write down the names of as many of your nurses and other personnel as possible. After you are home from your stay, they also appreciate your cards and letters.

- Be sure that the language, dietary, and cultural issues provided to the hospital are known to the floor staff as well.

- Familiarize yourself with your baseline vital signs, and record this baseline for use in comparing later values for any change.

- For all lab draws or medication doses, or intravenous solutions, make sure that the staff member providing the service does an appropriate positive ID prior to starting the collection, drug, or IV. Identification should be with at least two items, preferably full name and medical record number.

- Keep track of all medicines prescribed for you in the hospital and check each attempted dose against the list of medications ordered. Since medications may change or the doses may be adjusted during the stay, this requires continual exchange of information with the nursing staff.

- Be sure to compare the list of prescribed medications with the patient's allergy list to verify that no potentially allergic medications have been inadvertently prescribed.

- Also pay attention to the prescribed medication interval or number of doses per day as well as the size of each dose to verify that the right medicines in the

right doses at the right intervals are being given.

- **For all infusion pump based intravenous infusions, ask the nurse setting up the pump to verify the rate of infusion and the planned length of the infusion prior to starting the pump.**

- **For all x-ray or other imaging studies, be sure that the staff confirms positive identification of the patient before taking them to the imaging department.**

- **For all procedures (catheter placement, chest tube placement, electrode placement, cardiology procedure, in-room biopsy, or other therapy), be sure that positive identification is confirmed prior to either performing the procedure or to moving the patient to the procedural area.**

- **For all meals or dietary orders, keep track of what type of diet the patient is on (for example NPO – nothing by mouth, clear liquids, full liquids, soft diet, full diet etc) and make sure that any meal or snack delivered to them is consistent with their ordered diet. An accidental feeding of the patient prior to surgery will delay the case since anesthesia does not do well on a full stomach.**

- **Before any surgery, make sure that the surgeon and the patient "mark the site" to avoid wrong site surgery.**

After Surgery or during illness

- Be sure that vital signs (pulse rate, respiration rate, blood pressure, temperature, and oxygen saturation) are monitored and that you note any substantial changes in these parameters. Increased or decreased blood pressure can be dangerous, and increased pulse rate, especially with lower blood pressure can indicate loss of volume and potentially shock. Patients have very different baseline values for many parameters. Check the pre-op blood pressure and pulse to use as a guideline to evaluate post op changes. Temperature and oxygen saturation vary less widely high or low temperature values and oxygen saturation values below 90% are cause for concern. Your first concern is that the patient's nurse is noting and paying attention to any significant changes in these values.

- If the nurse decides to call a physician or another nurse for a concern about the patient, make sure that there is a response in a reasonable period of time. No more than 30 minutes.

- Have the hospital's "Code H" number in case you need to call attention to your patient yourself.

- Once the patient is out of anesthesia and able to communicate, make sure that they are receiving sufficient pain medicine for their level of surgical pain.

- Do not allow the nurse to place the patient in restraints without a full and detailed assessment of their vital signs and condition.

- Be sure to follow all the above "in their room" precautions regarding identification for various activities, medications, etc. Imaging studies are generally not scheduled in the immediately post-op period with the possible exception of portable chest films done in the patient's room. If radiology is trying to move the post op patient to radiology, they may have the wrong patient.

- Be aware of the patient's blood group and type (A,B,O,AB are "groups", Rh negative or positive are "types"). And be sure that any transfusion pays attention to the patient's group and type (note that often patients do not receive exactly the same blood type as their own native type. "O" blood may be given safely to any blood group patient, and often males or older females beyond childbearing age are switched to a "positive" from a "negative" type with no adverse impact. Also AB patients may safely receive either AB, A, B, or O groups).

Special Precautions

- **Blood thinners (anticoagulants)** Whether the patient was on warfarin at home, or was placed on warfarin in the hospital, be sure that there is a daily clotting time or "protime" drawn.

- **Other blood thinners, such as heparin, may or may not have requirements for laboratory monitoring depending on the type of medicine, the dose, and the duration of therapy.**

- **In all cases, if you notice the patient bleeding from blood draw sites, gums, or any other area such as their surgical wound, alert the nurse immediately.**

Before Discharge

- Be sure that the patient has prescriptions for all medications that have been added or temporarily prescribed for recovery.

- Be sure that there are clear, written, directions on what former medications to resume taking, discontinue, or change doses of following discharge.

- Be sure that there are clear, written, directions on any dietary restrictions or recommendations following discharge.

- Be sure that there are clear, written, directions on any restrictions on activity or travel following discharge. In some cases, prolonged travel by car has been catastrophic in the post-operative phase

- **Be sure that there are clear, written, directions on handling, output, and planned duration of any drains or catheters still in the patient at discharge.**

- **Be sure that there are clear written directions on any new medical equipment needed after discharge. Examples would include oxygen equipment, etc.**

- **Be sure to have a set of follow up directions, either an appointment with the physician or a plan to set up a follow up appointment.**

- **Be sure to have written information on how to contact the physician, surgeon, and their on-call group in the event of problems after discharge.**

After Discharge

- Be sure that the patient receives their medication as prescribed, including both new or "temporary" medicines as well as the former medications to be resumed.

- Be sure that the patient continues to show stable vital signs and lack of bleeding or unexpected discharges.

- Be sure that the patient follows the direction on activity provided before discharge.

- Be sure that the patient progresses in their activities, and diet according to the physicians' plan.

- Be sure to monitor any bleeding or drainage from wounds, catheters, or drains still present.

- **Be prepared to call the physician's office or their call group if there is any significant concern regarding the patient's condition or progress.**

www.ingramcontent.com/pod-product-compliance
Lightning Source LLC
Chambersburg PA
CBHW072322290526
45794CB00002B/725